Facing Fate with Faith

Bible Companion
for Those Affected by Cancer

JANET GASTON

with

DEBRA MCLEAN

WESTBOW
PRESS

WestBow Press books may be ordered through booksellers or by contacting:

WestBow Press
A Division of Thomas Nelson
1663 Liberty Drive
Bloomington, IN 47403
www.westbowpress.com
1-(866) 928-1240

ISBN: 978-1-4497-9924-3 (sc)
ISBN: 978-1-4497-9925-0 (e)

Library of Congress Control Number: 2013911592

Printed in the United States of America.

WestBow Press rev. date: 9/6/2013

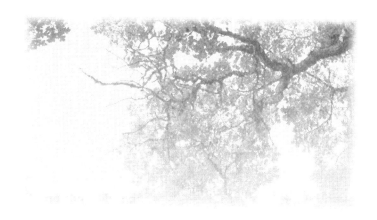

DEDICATION

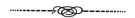

"Facing Fate with Faith" was written for the glory of my Heavenly Father, and to His son Jesus Christ. As you read this book, may the Holy Spirit touch your heart and life, and turn you towards the Holy Bible for further inspiration.

"Facing Fate with Faith—A Bible Companion for Cancer Patients and Survivors" is dedicated to all those who face a cancer diagnosis, whether they are currently undergoing treatment or are many years from diagnosis.

I am deeply grateful for the dedicated medical community who serve cancer patients, and whose lives are touched in the process.

My humble prayer is that pastors, chaplains, preachers and those who minister to the people under their spiritual care will also find "Facing Fate with Faith" a useful tool in reaching out with compassion to those affected by cancer—the patient and their caregivers. Perhaps it will help in answering some of the difficult questions that come up when walking this unexpected path.

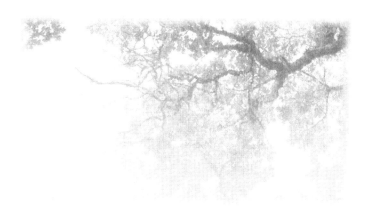

FOREWORD

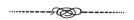

Hearing the words "you have cancer" is a pivotal moment in the life of anyone, forcing one to face death, which in turn brings all other aspects of your life into sharp focus. When survival is your motivation, all of life's other distractions become just that—distractions. Life becomes increasingly precious, ironically, because of death. Of course, life is by definition a terminal condition, but most of us spend years unconsciously believing that we will somehow escape this reality.

With the uncertainty that cancer brings, and the very real possibility of death, many people choose to pare down their lives to only what is most important. For many, there is a renewed focus on family and close, supportive friends; for some it might include distancing themselves or even ending unhealthy relationships; many re-envision their careers; some finally have the courage to pursue a passion; many question the role of faith in their lives; and many define (or refine) their life's mission. The answers that emerge from this journey are as varied and personal as the people involved.

The role of faith in Janet's life is central to her very being, and she has put together a series of devotionals that speak from her cancer journey—they address peace and acceptance; strength and perseverance; hope and love. For those who read this book, I hope you will find comfort, as well as a connection to survivors who came before you and those who will come after you; for those who have conquered this disease; for those who have not; and for those who continue to fight.

Wishing you strength, peace, and most of all love.

Your Survivor Sister since July 2006,
Lora Woodruff

"A beautiful testimony of how our Heavenly Father heals at all turns of life. A woman's fierce courage facing adversity. A mother's devotion to her children. A wife's dedication to her husband who fights beside her. Powerful and awesome in every way. Laughter, tears, happy, sad, learning, appreciation, humble . . . I experienced all of these feelings."

Jennifer Steen-Reavis,
Survivor and Nurse Navigator

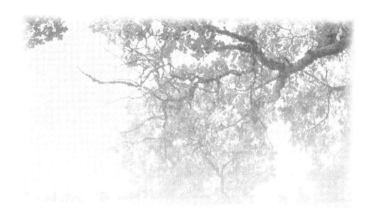

PREFACE

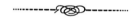

The purpose of this Bible companion that has made its way into your hands is to provide words of light, encouragement and comfort to those facing a diagnosis of cancer. I want to point your attention to the Bible to find truths upon which you can rest assured. It is my hope and prayer that regardless of the stage or progression of your disease, as you study the scriptures and read these devotions you will find messages from God intended just for you.

I have long felt called to write this book, both from a constant internal nagging voice, and because I have been uniquely placed in a position to experience cancer from many different vantage points.

My first cancer experience came in July 2006, when I was diagnosed with breast cancer. My son was only seven months old. In September of that same year, I joined a support group for young survivors of breast cancer. We have many strong, brave and insightful women in our group. After fighting bravely for as long as they were able, we lost three of our members to cancer.

I enjoyed two and a half years of treatment-free time after finishing my breast cancer journey. In June 2009, I gave birth to my daughter, another beautiful gift from God. When she was just a few months old, my family and I entered an incredible testing period.

In August 2009, my mother was diagnosed with breast cancer.

In September 2009, I was diagnosed with ovarian cancer.

In November 2009, my sister was diagnosed with ovarian cancer and continues to fight the disease.

In addition to immediate family members, my mother-in-law is also a cancer survivor and has had multiple occurrences. My father-in-law has battled prostate cancer. And my grandmother had two occurrences of breast cancer before finally succumbing to cancer at the age of 90. Her mother, my great-grandma, died at age 38 from breast cancer. Cancer is not a stranger here.

After treatment for ovarian cancer in 2009, I had almost two years of good health. In February 2012, I learned that my ovarian cancer had relapsed, and I continue to fight the disease today. So to say cancer has been inside of and all around me is an understatement. How did my family and I make it through these terrible trying times? We have made it so far because we have not gone alone. The God of comfort has been with us every step of the way. In the midst of every storm, we can find comfort in the Word of God and the presence of His Holy Spirit. I did just that, and I want to show you what helped me, so that it might help you too. Please use this book as a starting place, but ultimately, delve deep into the Bible for yourself, as this is where you can truly saturate your soul with God's love. Yes, God, our Awesome Creator and Savior, wrote us love letters.

God is a giver of good gifts filled with love. He has given us this world to live in. He has given us life. He gave us His one and only son, Jesus Christ. God even allowed his son, Jesus, to suffer and die on the cross to wash away our sins. Through Christ, we have the gift of eternal life. We also have the gift of the Holy Spirit—the greatest comforter and counselor ever. Jesus says in John 14:16 (KJV), "And I will pray the Father, and He shall give you another Comforter, that He may abide with you forever." In His Holy Bible God has given us love letters and encouragement on how to live through the difficult times we face. As we experience our trials, we learn how to comfort others in their similar trials. This brings us healing as we share in the hope.

> Praise be to the God and Father of our Lord Jesus Christ, the Father of compassion and the God of all comfort, who comforts us in all our troubles, so that we can comfort those in any trouble with the comfort we ourselves have received from God.
> 2 Corinthians 1:3 (NIV)

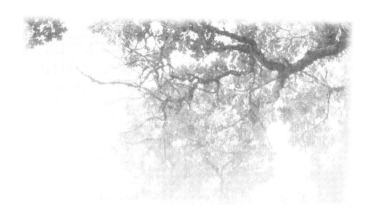

ACKNOWLEDGMENT

I am sincerely thankful for my editor, Cary Goldberg, for all of the time and wisdom she invested in this book with me. She has been my angel in so many ways. She took a very rough first draft from me that was half journaling, half book, and helped me mold it into this finished product. I am in her debt for all the versions she reviewed for me. I am also grateful for her encouragement in completing this project. In the process, she helped me develop into a better writer. I am grateful to my sister, Debra McLean, for her assistance in writing and rewriting this book. Debbie provided her own insights and polished this manuscript by using her logical mind to give the book a smooth flow.

"What are you trying to say here?" she often asked me. "Then let's write that." ☺ I am thankful to others who previewed this book, and encouraged me along the way: Lora, Cindy, Nicole, Linda, Don, Amanda, Lise, Donna, Jennifer and Coral. To Pastor Grant Knepper, thank you for going over the manuscript for Biblical soundness. Thank you for your great ideas and insights too. I am thankful to all of the people who have helped my family through our cancer battles over the last seven years. You prayed for us, brought us meals, bread, coffee, cookies and other treats; cleaned our house, did our laundry and dishes, fed, held and diapered our babies, read to our children, encouraged us with phone calls, visits, cards; and all the while reminded us of the love of God. We are forever grateful for your acts of kindness. I am blessed to have a wonderful husband who has always stood by my side, weathering the storms. Jason, you are a wonderful husband, and I love you. I am grateful for the blessing of our two beautiful children, Gabriel and Amelia. As babies and small children, Gabriel and Amelia, you brought me such comfort and inspiration to keep fighting. I love you to Heaven and back. Most importantly, I am grateful for our Heavenly Father, His son Jesus Christ, and the Holy Spirit for their indescribable gifts!

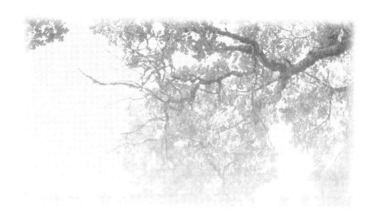

INTRODUCTION

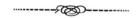

When you received the initial diagnosis of cancer, what did you do? How did you feel?

When I received my first cancer diagnosis, I felt like someone had opened the door to a very dark hallway and pushed me to start walking. I did not know what to do or where to go. My whole world turned upside down, and I felt so alone. My infant son was there, and I was trying not to fall apart in front of him.

Then I picked up the phone and called a friend who gave me a dose of perspective, saying she knew I would make it through, and at least it was not my child. Next, I called my husband, and he came home with a huge hug for me. His presence grounded me back in the moment, and I was no longer physically alone. I still had this cancer diagnosis and moments where I felt set apart from those who love me. Yet into my life shined rays of light and hope given to me from a very loving Heavenly Father. God reached out, hugged me through my husband, and gave me the strength to fight and live. God reached out to me with support, help and love through my family and friends.

During Bible readings throughout my cancer journeys, our loving Heavenly Father also opened my eyes to understand and embrace His words, reaching me with His loving grace. Meditating on certain verses and realizing deeper meanings from them was helpful. God's word is available to reach out in love to all of us. You too can face a cancer diagnosis with faith as you unlock the secrets of the scripture to find hope, comfort, grace, peace, and reassurance as you draw closer to the heart of God.

Since initially I had a complete response to my chemotherapy treatments, I feel so richly blessed by our Heavenly Father. I always knew he had the power to heal me. I did not always know what He would chose to do, heal me or not heal me, but I knew it was completely up to His will. The power to heal is definitely there. I'd like to think that the many, many, many prayers said on my behalf, asking the King to heal me, may have persuaded Him. Yet I know others out there were lifted up in prayer that for reasons we will never understand were not fully healed. We have to completely trust the Good Lord that He knows what He is doing. <u>WE</u> may not know, <u>but HE DOES</u>.

Blessed be the name of the Lord. His name is always worthy of our praise.

We must remember that even though we are cancer patients or survivors, cancer is not our identity. We are not the disease. Our identities are secure as children of God, created in His image. To affirm this, we can look at the beginning of the Bible in Genesis and read about the creation of Adam and Eve. Psalm 139:14, "I will praise thee; for I am fearfully and wonderfully made: marvelous are thy works; and that my soul knoweth right well."(KJV)

Though we face the fate of dealing with this terrible disease, we are not alone. Jesus has given us the ultimate counselor—the Holy Spirit. We have His written words found in the Holy Bible that give us the tools and encouragement to face our fates with faith. Romans 8 is a wonderful chapter for giving us Christian assurance. It reminds us that we are adopted children of our Heavenly Father. That we have been given a spirit of sonship, and not of fear.

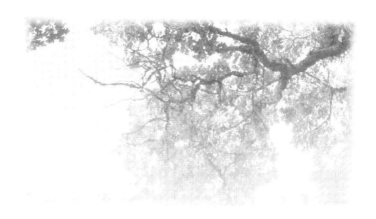

TABLE OF CONTENTS

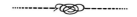

Lesson 1:   Fear & Worry 1

Lesson 2:   Praying for Healing 7

Lesson 3:   Serving 12

Lesson 4:   Strength & Perseverance for the Journey 17

Lesson 5:   Rest 25

Lesson 6:   Trust 33

Lesson 7:   Perspective 39

Lesson 8:   Suffering 43

Lesson 9:   Sorrow, Loss & Loneliness 47

Lesson 10: Gratitude 50

Lesson 11: Wisdom 56

Lesson 12: Facing Death & Dying with Hope 60

Epilogue 67

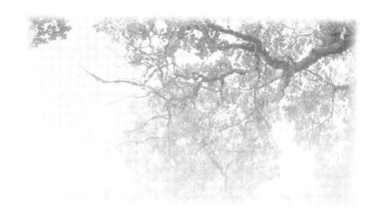

LESSON 1

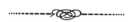

Fear & Worry

Isaiah 41:10: "So do not fear, for I am with you; do not be dismayed, for I am your God. I will strengthen you and help you; I will uphold you with my righteous right hand." (NIV)

My aunt sent me this verse during my breast cancer treatments in a beautiful card. I kept it in my Bible and referred to it often. It is an example of God's beautiful promises. When we lean on Him to take care of us, there is no reason to fear.

Listen to Jesus' words on worry. He tells us many times in the Bible not to be afraid. Here are a few words

He says, taken from Matthew 6:25 (KJV): "Therefore I say unto you, Take no thought for your life, what ye shall eat, or what ye shall drink; nor yet for your body, what ye shall put on. Is not the life more than meat, and the body more than raiment?"

I had heard this passage several times before cancer. I could not wrap my head around it and believe it fully. To tell me not to worry was like telling me not to breathe. Until cancer. Then when faced with the realization that I really might not be breathing in the near future, the passages from St. Matthew 6:25-34 and St. Luke 12:22-34 helped me realize what a waste of time worry is. Especially Jesus's words in verse 27 which point out that worrying does not add time to our lives, and in verse 34 that point out it is best to take one day at a time and not worry about tomorrow. I grabbed onto these verses like life preservers. After a diagnosis of cancer, the whole passage had new meaning for me.

I remember one day about a week after my diagnosis and before I was starting treatment where I just went and sat in my closet to hide and feel despondent. I was caught by my husband, who lovingly scolded me, so it was only a matter of minutes that I spent in the closet. There is no hiding for the mother of an eight-month-old baby. I learned there were more constructive things to do with my time than sitting and worrying.

Then I reread the passage from Jesus in Matthew 6 and his advice on worrying. As I read Jesus' words, "Who of you by worrying can add a single hour to his life?" (verse 27, NIV), I suddenly heard the humor and irony in his voice and wondered if that was his original tone. I realized that sitting in the closet feeling awful was not adding time to my life, it was only taking it away. To sit and wonder what my son was going to do if I died, or my husband, or if the cancer was spreading, or if I would make it through treatments, or about anything at all—the time I spent worrying and sitting in fear was just lost time. I had to ask myself, is this how I want to spend the time I do have, wallowing in negative emotions like fear and worry? During cancer treatments, each day certainly does have enough trouble of its own! Troubling side effects, confusing information to process, appointments to go to, being poked at, prodded, tested, lacking the energy to do all that needs to be done, calls to insurance companies to fight over who is paying and how much—it was all too much!

I realized it was much better to follow Jesus' advice in verse 34 and take one day at a time. His words set me free from the worry and fear, giving me permission to focus on and enjoy each moment and each day as it comes. I learned it was much healthier to focus on the present and to take one day at a time. Will you let His words set you free too?

I encourage you to read Matthew 6:25-34 and the Gospel of Luke in chapter 12 and ask God what He wants you to see and understand from Jesus' wise words on worry. Both passages from Matthew and Luke emphasize that our Heavenly Father knows what we need and He will provide it. This is a comforting realization that God is taking care of us. In the midst of our difficulties, He is there looking out for us. He is with us. We need not worry. We can trust Him. At times we may feel like He is not there, but He is.

When you get rid of fear and worry, like with all bad habits, you will have extra time so replace it with something positive. What could be more positive than praising our Lord? I challenge you to replace fear and worry with praise. Try humming or singing a song.

One of my favorite passages that has helped me get through difficult times even before cancer, is from Philippians 4:8 (NLT)

> And now, dear brothers and sisters, let me say one more thing as I close this letter. Fix your thoughts on what is true and honorable and right. Think about things that are pure and lovely and admirable.

Think about things that are excellent and worthy of praise.

So don't think about the cancer. Think about the beautiful smile on your child's face. Think about him learning to walk. Think about the beautiful morning sunlight dancing off of the grass and dew. Think about how many people love you and are providing help. Think about having the strength to go for a walk today, even though it was shorter than you used to take. Think about who came over and did your laundry so you could rest. Think about the kind people who bring dinner over once a week. Think about your friends' lives and the positive things happening for them. Think about babies yet to be born. Think about how well you handled a chemotherapy treatment. Think about how you can constructively use the time during your treatments, i.e., by taking knitting, scrapbooking, sewing, writing, reading, listening to music. Think about what brings joy into your life and start doing it—watch humorous shows. Plant a seed and watch it grow. If you play a musical instrument, continue to do so. And PRAISE GOD FOR ALL OF IT.

Worry's partner is fear and fear is definitely an active emotion for us as cancer patients. Fear of the unknown, fear of the treatments, fear of side effects, fear of the future and all the other garbage that goes with cancer. When we have thoughts of fear and anxiousness, it is important to recognize them and then deal with them constructively. Be ready to know where to take them. God is before us and beside us and we can take those fears to Him, knowing he will never leave us or forsake us. The Lord is near and ready to listen. Philippians chapter 4, verses 5-7 reassures us of this. Fear does not do good things for us or for others. Try to avoid it by asking God to fill you with His love, and His peace that surpasses our understanding. When times are bleak and discouraging, we can rely on God's promises. He is there to lift us up every day in the midst of our despair.

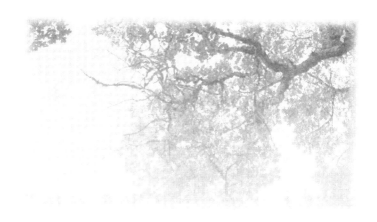

LESSON 2

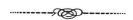

Praying for Healing

Prayer is an important part of the healing process. There is a certain comfort in knowing that others are praying for you, so ask people to pray for you. Be specific in your requests and pray for yourself. When I was first diagnosed with cancer, it was hard to come up with words to speak to God on my own. Fortunately, God directed me to the words to pray within the Holy Scriptures.

My first experience with cancer started on a Friday with a call from my gynecologist telling me I had breast cancer. That Sunday, my mom insisted that she and my dad join my family at church. I had left a message or two with my pastor but had not gotten to speak with him yet about my cancer diagnosis. He had been traveling out of town. We sat in the service and listened to a sermon that seemed to be custom made for us—two stories of Jesus healing two different women in the Holy Gospels. My mom took it as a sign. I found my prayer. The passages from the sermon were: Mark 5:21-43 (NIV) and Luke 8:40-56 (NIV). One story is of a woman who had been sick and suffering for many years. She is healed after she touches Jesus' cloak, because she had faith in his power to heal. In the second story, Jesus brings back to life a girl who had recently died, restoring the child to full health. These examples of Jesus healing when many would say hope was gone are quite inspirational. I took Mark 5:34 and wrote it as a prayer on a little strip of paper. I kept that strip of paper in my Bible throughout all my treatments. Whenever I came across it, I would pray these words: "Dear Jesus, please say to me like you said to the woman in Mark 5:34 (NIV), 'Daughter, your faith has healed you. Go in peace and be freed from your suffering.'" This was a pleading prayer, for sure, but it was my lifeline to God when the words did not come on my own. When we don't know what to pray we can always pray scripture.

Another scripture that I used as prayer is found in Psalm 30, verses 2-3 and 8-12 (KJV). I had this one handwritten on my refrigerator for a long time. Verse 2 (NIV) read, "O Lord my God, I cried unto thee, and thou hast healed me." The other verses ask what benefit could come from my death? If I am alive I can work to bring Him glory and praise. This was my plea for why I should continue to live. I identified with this passage because I did not understand what gain could come from my death. I had a baby to take care of and young family to live for. I felt strongly that there was still work to do for the Lord. I was pleading for his help and healing.

Psalm 30 describes what the Lord does and how we should respond. In Verse 11, the psalmist tells us God changed things for him. And what am I willing to give in return? I should proclaim His faithfulness and praise His name! See Verse 12, "that my heart may sing to you and not be silent. O Lord my God, I will give you thanks forever."(NIV) Even in our suffering when we spend time in prayer we can experience a shift in mindset. When we talk to God, cry out to Him in whatever we are going through He will help us. Through prayer, we can ask God to turn our wailing into dancing. We can find that there is meaning in our situations even though we do not see what it is directly. We can praise God even when our current circumstances feel helpless. Praying does not mean that healing from cancer will come. God does not promise that if we pray enough we will be free from disease or hardships. He has the power to heal us. He may heal us, He may not, but prayer does provide healing for our soul. We can be sure that God hears us when we cry out to Him. Psalm 66:19 (KJV) states: "but verily God hath heard me; he hath attended to the voice of my prayer." I know for me, just being heard, even when things do not change, makes me feel better emotionally.

God certainly has the power to heal. In Matthew 8:5-13(NIV), we see a wonderful example of Jesus' healing power. Jesus heals the Centurion's servant. This man gives us a good example of faith. He did not even need Jesus to go to his servant. Just say the word Jesus, and my servant will be healed, he said (verse 8). He recognized Jesus' authority and understood Christ's power. There was no doubt in the Centurion's mind what Jesus was capable of doing. All he needed was for Jesus to say the word. And Jesus does. When the Centurion goes home he finds his servant was healed.

Another example of Jesus' healing power is a well-known story found in John 11:17-44 (NIV), where Jesus raises his friend, Lazarus, from the dead. In this amazing story, by the time Jesus had reached the town where Mary, Martha and Lazarus lived, Lazarus had already been dead for four days. That did not stop Jesus. After Mary and Martha appealed to him, falling at his feet and crying, Jesus went to where the body lay. After praying to our Heavenly Father, Jesus called out in a loud voice, "Lazarus, come out!" and lo and behold, Lazarus did as Jesus told him, and he was alive again! It is obvious to me from these stories that Jesus was an incredible healing physician. Cancer can leave us with emotional, physical and spiritual scars. Yet we have the ultimate healer. If we let Him take away our pain, bitterness and emotional and spiritual scars, He will do it. God can heal in many ways. When we take our requests for healing to the Lord in prayer, God may answer—giving us healing to our physical bodies through the works of modern medicine and medical professionals, healing hands, or miracles or other ways. In some instances, we may not receive physical healing, but instead He heals our hearts and gives us peace. Our part is to pray and trust our Great Physician with our lives and souls. In the process, we grow in our faith.

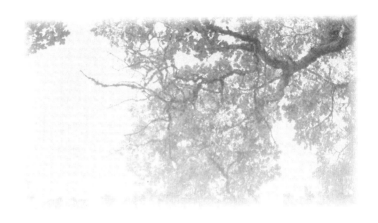

LESSON 3

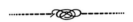

Serving

A cancer diagnosis causes most people to stop and analyze their lives. Are we really doing what we should? Are we who we want to be? We question our relationships, jobs and choices we have made. We search for meaning. What have we done? Is it enough? When I asked myself these searching questions, I found satisfaction in my decision to be a stay-at-home mom. After my illness, I wanted to help in the community outside of my home. I found the ability to give back and to serve others offered me a wonderful outlet and a path toward healing. We can serve others in some way, encouraging them, reaching out in love and compassion, reminding those that are grieving and sick that they are never alone.

While doing things for other people, my focus shifted from my own health concerns to the recipient's needs. Changing my perspective stopped the depression spiral that can occur with cancer. Instead of wallowing in self-pity, hope bloomed as seeds of service were planted. In times of remission and good health, serving others helps the healing process. This is our chance to give the help back we received when we were sick. The Bible says, "Cast thy bread upon the waters: for thou shall find it after many days." Ecclesiastes 11:1 (KJV). When you give to others all around you, much shall be given back to you.

Jesus said in John 12:26 (KJV), "If any man serve me, let him follow me; and where I am, there shall also my servant be: if any man serve me, him will my Father honour." After speaking these words, Jesus offers an excellent example of serving for his disciples, and it is recorded in the Gospel of John, chapter 13, verses 1-17. In this passage, Jesus washes his disciples' feet. It was just before the Passover feast. They had been traveling around in sandals and their feet were very dirty. Washing feet was a servant's job in those days. Jesus, the Son of God, was their leader, and yet, He humbled himself and cleaned their feet. When Peter asked if Jesus really was going to clean his feet, Christ insisted. Peter was surprised that he would take that lowly job, but Jesus emphasized that it was very important for him to do, and said, "Unless I wash you, you have no part with me." (Verse 8b—NIV) Jesus washed their feet to show His love and the importance of serving. Afterwards, he asked them if they understood his actions. He tells them to follow His example. Once the disciples understood that they were called to humbly reach out in love to others for the Lord, and they did as He asked, they would be blessed. What greater incentive is there for service than the promise of blessings from our Lord and Savior, Jesus Christ?

I have seen so many blessings come into my life. When I give to others, it certainly comes back, sometimes tenfold. And when others give to me, I want to give back to them. A woman in our support group wanted to help someone. This kind-hearted woman is a breast cancer survivor. When she was diagnosed, she was in a hard situation, a single mom, jobless. The founder of our support group took her under her wing and helped her through, restoring hope and providing what her family needed at the time. This woman now has a great job, good health and is paying forward the favors. During treatments after my third cancer diagnosis I was the recipient of her generosity. Receiving her gift encouraged me and made me feel worthwhile. When my health allows, I like to look for opportunities to pay it forward.

My second battle with cancer, in large part because it was linked with watching both my mom and sister undergo cancer treatment at the same time, led me into a very sad place. I spent a lot of time in sorrow. And there was much grief too. Yet part of what helped me get through those dark days was to find little things I could do for others. This forced me to stay in the "land of the living" and to find something good about each day.

In 2 Corinthians 9:6-8 we are reminded, when we willingly and generously give, we will reap generously. As cancer patients (and survivors) we may think we do not have much to give. But God makes sure we do. See verse 8 (NIV): "And God is able to make all grace abound to you, so that in all things at all times, having all that you need, you will abound in every good work." Through our cancer experiences, we have wisdom and insights we can share with others about life and about the dying process. Though physically we are limited in energy, at times we can still be a support to each other and to our families. There is great healing in helping others. The old saying, "It is easier to give than receive" is true. When we are battling cancer, most of the time we find ourselves on the receiving end. Sometimes we need to wait until we are finished with treatments and a year down the recovery path before we feel we can start giving back. You need time to heal. Jesus received loving care from one of His friends shortly before His death. In Mark chapter 14, we read about the woman anointing Jesus with oil, bringing Him comfort. Jesus said, verse 6 (KJV), "Let her alone; why trouble ye her? She hath wrought a good work on me." You can read the story again in Matthew 26:6-13 and St. John 12:1-8.

When we are battling cancer, we need help. Yet, if we think creatively, we can endeavor to be on the giving end at times too. Calling someone to chat or sharing with others from our abundance are simple ways to serve. It is the thought and the willingness to serve that makes a difference in someone else's life. We can rest assured that our attempts at service are acceptable in God's eyes because of 2 Corinthians 8:12 (KJV): "For if there be first a willing mind, it is accepted according to that a man hath, and not according to that he hath not." When we have the desire for service, God may provide the means. If we learn to follow Jesus' example, as he said in Matthew 20:28 (NLT), "For even I, the Son of Man, came here not to be served but to serve others, and to give His life a ransom for many," we can start to understand the importance of serving and how we can apply it in our lives.

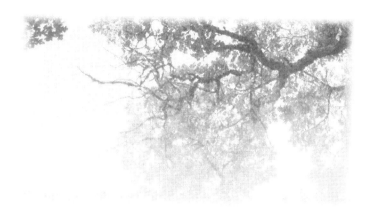

LESSON 4

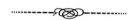

Strength & Perseverance for the Journey

The cancer journey can be very long and trying. We need strength and perseverance to continue the fight. I understand this, because I have fought cancer three different times in more than six years. With each occurrence, I find the need for renewed strength and perseverance. As I am currently battling cancer a fourth time, I often wish I could give up. Yet my children's beautiful faces encourage me to keep trying. Hugs from my daughter, interesting conversations with my son, and my husband still needs me too. I cannot desert them. Yet how can I keep going week after week to receive the medicine that could save my life, yet makes me tired and sick with side effects? The only way I can keep going is through Christ's strength. I have been given so much to carry; it is only by leaning on His strength that I can keep going.

The journey is very hard. There are many tears, fears and trials along the way. How do we make it? We can stand and rest on the promises of God. We can remember that God is able! We may not be able, but God has promised to be there to comfort and strengthen us. We can trust in Him. Paul tells of his vision of the Lord in 2 Corinthians 12:1-10 (KJV). In verse 9 Jesus tells him that God's grace is sufficient for him. His power is made perfect in weakness. In verse 10 (KJV) Paul gives us a different perspective on our weakness: "Therefore I take pleasures in infirmities, in reproaches, in necessities, in persecutions, in distresses for Christ's sake: For when I am weak, then am I strong." When we remember that God is all-powerful and that he blesses us with undeserved love, we can shake our discouragement, difficulties and trials. When we focus on Him and his greatness, our anger can melt away. Our broken hearts begin to heal, and we find strength flow into us from the Holy Spirit.

Here is an excerpt from Debbie's blog:

At the radiation department I had my radiation set up. That went fast and easy. They laid a rubbery mesh thing over my face. It felt like a damp wash cloth. I think it is some sort of plastic, when it dries it hardens and forms the mask. The technicians made some marks on it and did a quick CT scan of my head. I kept my eyes closed and thought of Matthew West's song, "Strong Enough", in particular the part that goes, 'I can do all things, through Christ who gives me strength.' They asked me how I was doing and I tried to say "okay" and then realized that the mask is so tight that you can't move your mouth to talk. And then it was over, I got off the table, and waited for my radiation oncologist. Thank you God for being strong enough for me to give you this too.

I am starting radiation on Tuesday. Kind of looking forward to it. Bring it on, let's do this. I plan to spend the time in prayer and thanksgiving. I should be done by the end

of the following week. Originally I thought
I could do them all in a row, but now it
sounds like I have to do it every other day,
so it will take two weeks instead of one.

Debbie leaned on God to see her through her brain
radiation treatments. I saw her mask and it looked like
something out of a horror movie. I am not happy my
sister had to go through this. If it was up to me, she
would never have had to endure that for two weeks. I
do not see why this was a part of her journey. Yet I am
not in control and God sees what we do not see. His
ways are so much higher than our ways. We can trust
God is working all of this into a beautiful masterpiece.
It may not turn out, and most likely will not all turn
out the way we may want it to. But there is a great work
He is orchestrating through our pain and suffering. He
is working on it for His Glory. And through it all, He
is instructing us on how to reach out to others with His
love and grace. When Debbie heard my cancer had come
back once again, she wrote the following in her blog:

I was glad that I read this the day before:
"He will have no fear of bad news; his heart
is steadfast, trusting in the Lord." Psalm
112:7 (NIV). This was also helpful with all

the craziness that is happening in the world today. We don't have to fear bad news, we can trust in God and that He is in control. We can't see the big picture, but we know there is one and that we are part of it. God continues to give me His peace. This is a crazy journey and I don't know all the places it will lead but I know God is faithful always. He will never leave us or forsake us.

Throughout the scriptures, God encourages us to persevere. One example is in Hebrews 10:36 (NLT): "Patient endurance is what you need now, so you will continue to do God's will. Then you will receive all that he has promised."

Romans 5:3-5 (NIV), also encourages us to persevere in our suffering, because those experiences help us develop character and hope. This passage also reminds us that God loves us and gives us the Holy Spirit. The Holy Spirit is our ultimate comforter. When we are going through cancer, we need this comfort, hope, and love. May you find examples of it throughout the Holy Scriptures.

When we trust in His promises, we can stand firm despite our circumstances. The goal is to get to the point where you trust in Him no matter what. Recall the promises made by God to us in our baptism. We are a child of God and he holds us firmly in the palm of His hand. We need to make the conscious decision to persist in this hope without exception. If we keep going towards the goal, God promises to sustain us. 2 Corinthians 4:16 (NLT), encourages us: "That is why we never give up. Though our bodies are dying, our spirits are being renewed every day." Ideally, we can feel daily renewed by reading the scriptures, praying and recalling the promises made by God in baptism. However, in reality, there were days the feelings of hopelessness were so overwhelming I could not see past my own pain to read the scriptures and find the words to pray. In those times, I tried to keep my chin up and quietly trust that God would see me through. Other days I cried out in anger and pain. At times, I found the strength to behave well, and at other times, not so much. When I did make the time to be with God and ask for His peace I found he filled me with His strength and helped me through the day's challenges. Often this encouragement and strength came through another person's timely kindnesses. Small acts of kindness, such as a phone call, home-baked cookies, flowers, or a hug were ways God used other people to uplift me.

James encourages us to look at difficult times in our lives differently than most of the world would. In the first chapter of the book of James, he says to, "consider it PURE JOY whenever you face trials of many kinds" James 1:2 (NIV). In verses 3-4 he tells us the testing of our faith develops perseverance. Faith is tested during our difficult times, or trials in life. Our trials help us mature and develop. Without trials our faith can become stagnant. I found that my trials with cancer pushed a much more aggressive growth in faith then I would have experienced without them. It forced me to trust in God for what we needed, (help with my babies and taking care of my home, etc.). During these experiences, I found myself getting to know God better. He challenged me to rest on the belief that He is good, despite circumstances, and that He would provide for us. The first time I was diagnosed, I did not know how or if I would survive. But God was faithful, seeing me and my family through it and I was healed. I thought it would not happen again, at least for a long time. The second diagnosis of cancer came just three years later. I did not know what the outcome would be, but, once again, God healed me. When the third diagnosis came I recalled James' verse about "considering it pure joy." While I might not have pure joy all the time, I had joy in my heart, because I knew God was faithful to sustain me. I knew that with each of these trials I had grown in trust and faith, maturing and developing, and that this trial would also bring about perseverance and hope.

In James 1:12 (NIV), we are reminded we are blessed when we persevere under trial.

Christ also understands our suffering and brings us comfort. 2 Corinthians 1:5-6 (NIV), summarizes how with Christ we suffer, receive comfort and develop patient endurance. We do not suffer alone. With Christ's comfort we can persevere, i.e., develop patient endurance while we suffer. We can rest assured that through this suffering, God's gift of salvation still prevails, and that He has never left our side.

In 2 Corinthians 6:3-10 (NIV) Paul reminds us that as servants of God we are going to run into all kinds of hardships and trials. Cancer is definitely at least one of them. We are going to feel that we are at our wit's end and there is nothing left for us to give, that we might just collapse into a puddle on the floor, or feel like a Mack truck has hit us. I know I have felt that way many times during my cancer journeys.

Remember in 2 Corinthians 12:8-9 (NIV), Paul tells us that he had an ongoing trial that he asked the Lord to take away. Yet the Lord chose to leave it there, because God's glory is shown through our weakness. Even though He may not take away our trials or answer our requests how we think He should, His grace is sufficient and we can rely on Him to stay with us throughout our journey.

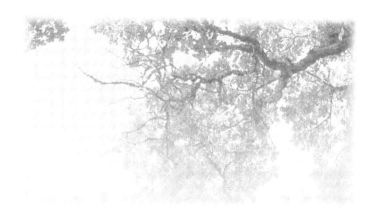

LESSON 5

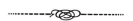

Rest

Fighting cancer is often exhausting. In my original diagnosis and each time I faced a return of cancer, I have experienced this exhaustion physically, emotionally, mentally, and spiritually. At times, we feel we may not be able to go on because of the extreme exhaustion in one or more aspects of life. Though our bodies lay in exhaustion, our minds might continue racing on, keeping us from getting the rest and sleep we need. How do we turn off these whirling minds? How do we get the rest we so desperately need? I have faced these questions repeatedly.

During these difficult times, you can receive rest from the Lord. God calls us to rest in Him. To get away from the fear, sorrow, and grief is the goal. We can come to Him in our raw pain and yell if we want to. Jesus offers to calm the waters inside us, as documented in the book of Matthew when He said,

> Come to me, all you who are weary and burdened, and I will give you rest. Take my yoke upon you and learn from me, for I am gentle and humble in heart and you will find rest for your souls. For my yoke is easy and my burden is light. Matthew 11:28-30 (NIV)

I find such comfort in these words. We can leave our burdens at the cross. We can give them to Jesus and replace them with a lighter load. He is willing to take our burdens away. He takes care of us. For us cancer patients, the stillness and rest we often seek is for our souls. Jesus offers us this rest.

Corrie Ten Boom, who hid Jews during World War II and wound up in a concentration camp herself for her efforts, wrote the book, "The Hiding Place." In this book she tells of a time when she was a child and her father taught her the lesson that some things were not meant to be carried by a child. Using his heavy suitcase as an example, when she was unable to make it budge, he told her he was there to carry it for her. Many years later, Corrie Ten Boom applied this lesson when she was in the concentration camp, by turning her heavy burdens to Jesus, saying, "Jesus, this is too heavy for me, will you carry this for me too?" In this way the horrors of the concentration camp were buffered for her by her Lord and Savior, Jesus Christ. Both my sister and I applied that example in our own journeys with cancer. Many times things are too hard to face on our own. We need loving friends and family willing to stand beside us. It is essential to know we have a Lord and Savior that carries our burdens for us. He reaches out to us through other people, placing our needs on their hearts. Through the Holy Spirit in action in other people, he comforts us, lightening our load.

During the nightmare of August 2009 through March 2010, I found the times that I turned it all over to the Lord, when I asked him to carry it for me, those were the times my load was lightened. Sometimes I would think, "How am I going to find the help I need for myself and my children during my surgeries? Or during my treatments?" Then I prayed for God to provide it. Hebrews 4:16 (KJV), "Let us therefore come boldly unto the throne of grace, that we may obtain mercy, and find grace to help in time of need." The next thing I knew, the phone would ring and someone was available to help me. At other times I felt sad and alone, and then the phone would ring with someone calling to say they were thinking of me. The help came from places I did not expect. So often, I felt His loving hand, His touch, and His words through other people. In Philippians 4, verses 19 and 20 Paul reminds us that our loving Heavenly Father meets our needs: "But my God shall supply all your need according to His riches in glory by Christ Jesus. Now unto God and our Father be glory for ever and ever. Amen." (KJV)

How we do find this rest? When we call upon Him and spend time in His Word, resting in His companionship, building our relationship with Him, we begin to find this rest. God calls us to rest in Him. We can look upon the beauty of the Lord and feel our tumults calmed in His presence. The Gospel gives a good example when Jesus calmed the storm for His disciples. Many times my family and I feel we have gone through storms too. It is a journey on the waves of life and until the storms pass we have to ride it out. We cannot control the storms and achieve peace on our own despite our best efforts to obtain it.

While fighting cancer there are times of rest. Between treatments, during remissions, while recovering from a surgery, and while receiving a chemotherapy treatment, one *must* rest. These may seem like times of unrest, but Jesus can give us a peace that surpasses our understanding. Only with this type of peace will we withstand the crashing waves. It is good to know we have a loving Savior we can look to, while the boat is rocking and tossing about. We have a Savior strong enough and with the authority to calm the wind and the waves. Sometimes He choses to calm the storm. Other times He lets the winds whip and the rains fall, and chooses to calm us on the inside instead.

God knows that rest is so important for our bodies that he set aside one day a week for us to do it. God rested himself on the seventh day of creation in Genesis 2:2-3 (KJV), "And on the seventh day God ended his work which he had made; and he rested on the seventh day from all his work which he had made. And God blessed the seventh day, and sanctified it: because that in it he had rested from all his work which God created and made."

So do not feel bad for resting. Instead, know that you are doing what you are designed to do. Try to enjoy it. The journeys through cancer battles have taught me to rest and look forward to times of rest and recovery and to balance them with times of activity.

There are so many benefits to learning to rest in God. Among them, is the peace that we can find through Him. Stop thinking we have to go, go, go, achieve, achieve, achieve. Instead, prioritize time with the Lord. Carve out a time daily to rest in God and allow His word to transform and heal us as we soak in His presence. Our anxiousness begins to melt away and we replace it with peace as we bask in the light of His presence. In my personal experiences, I find these moments when I am still and quiet to be incredible gifts. It is while I stopped doing and just listened that the insights were revealed. If I never slowed down, I would have missed out on those moments. Hebrews chapter 4 talks about a type of rest that is ours when we believe and hear His words in the Bible with faith.

The beginning of Psalm 91 1-2 tells us of the benefit of God's provision when we rest in Him. We can rest in Him as our hiding place. Feel free to pause and read that whole Psalm. It has wonderful images, including us under His wings, covered by His feathers, as if we were baby birds. When she was three, my daughter liked to pretend she was a baby bird with me. I would fly over bringing her food to pretend to put in her beak. We would make a cozy nest. I would sit on my "egg", waiting for it to hatch. We giggled with happiness.

We can find rest by waiting on the Lord. It is hard to be patient, especially when we do not know our long-term prognosis. We are reminded in Psalm 37:7a (KJV): "Rest in the Lord, and wait patiently for Him." Rest in God, spend time getting to know Him and faith in Him increases. He is glorified by it. Look at Psalm 46:10 (NIV), which says, "Be still, and know that I am God: I will be exalted among the nations, I will be exalted in the earth." With practice, stillness in God can become second nature to us.

Exodus 14:14 (KJV), "The Lord shall fight for you; and ye shall hold your peace." Moses tells the people this just before he receives instructions to part the Red Sea. There are storms behind and in front of them and God tells them that they only need to be still. He will take care of them. We can certainly rest in knowing the Lord is fighting for us too. Even when storms are going on around us, when we rest in God, He will sustain us. God is in control of the storms. As I stepped out of my car to walk into my oncology office to begin a third battle against cancer, knowing God was by my side gave me a peace and contentment in my soul. I thought of the Lord's words to Joshua after Moses' death, in the first chapter of the book of Joshua. Verse 9 (KJV), "Have I not commanded thee? Be strong and of a good courage; be not afraid, neither be thou dismayed: for the Lord thy God is with thee whithersoever thou goest." If I did not have God, my journey would have been impossible. Knowing He was right there with me in my most difficult hours made them endurable.

At times, I felt like an Israelite watching the Red Sea parting in front of me. Completing treatments and going into an NED—no evidence of disease—status is like crossing onto dry land. The tumultuous seas crash behind me, but I am safe, because my God rescued me! At other times, I felt like the Israelites stuck between a raging storm, sea and an army on their pursuit. I sympathize with the Israelites' terror, yet hear the words of Moses saying "BE STILL".

Being still and finding rest, especially in sleep is difficult at times, yet is important for our healing. Sleep can certainly be an issue at times for us when battling cancer, and even beyond. Our thoughts race while we lie in bed. Steroids given to help us process our treatments keep us awake. Changes to our bodies stop the normal sleep patterns. In Proverbs 3:21-26 God promises us no fear and sweet sleep. What a beautiful promise offered for us to embrace. Let us embrace this gift and learn to live in this rest, being still in His presence. How many cancer patients and survivors wish for peaceful sleep? Oh, that it could be so for us in our cancer journeys!

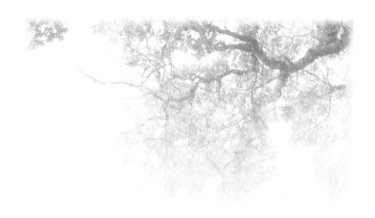

LESSON 6

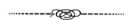

Trust

T rust can be a noun or verb. When used as a
noun, Webster's Dictionary defines trust as "the
assured reliance on the character, strength or truth
of someone or something." My husband said to me,
trust means not having to second guess someone, you
don't have to think twice. When it is a coworker, we
can trust their work, we don't feel we have to double
check everything they do. When it is a doctor or other
medical professional, we can trust they will do the
research, provide us with knowledge and guidance
to help us make the best decisions for our personal

medical situation. We can depend on them to be trustworthy.

Considering these definitions, we can ask ourselves if God is trustworthy. For the answer to that, (which is of course He is, by the way) let us look to the word He has given us—and the history of God's relation with His people—let's look to the Bible. We can start with stories of His promises to Abraham, to Isaac, and to Jacob. He fulfilled all of His promises to them and the ones He made to the Israelites. He fulfilled the ultimate promise of salvation, the original one mentioned in the beginning of the book of Genesis, when Adam and Eve sinned. He gave us His very own son, Jesus, sacrificed for our sins. Yes, we can answer with confidence that God is trustworthy. He kept His promises then and He keeps them now. We can rely on His character, strength and truth. This means that we can trust Him, even when we do not understand why or like the way things are going.

When Webster's Dictionary defines trust as a verb it is "to permit to stay or go or to do something without fear or misgiving, i.e., entrust or depend." We must have this type of trust in God so we can rely on Him, that He will make something beautiful from our lives. We should trust Him in all circumstances even when it strains our trust to its limits. He is the master weaver taking each piece of our lives and weaving the individual strands into a beautiful whole. We can trust in God. He wants the best for us. We cannot wrap our heads around and understand why things are going the way they are—especially when it is not how we would chose. Yet, we can know that His ways are so much higher than our ways. When we know God and His character, we trust who He is, not what is happening around us. The Bible often references Him as our rock, our refuge, our strength. Think of whom you trust most in your life. Are they a rock for you? Despite what is going on around you, can you depend on them to remain by your side and true to who they are? My husband has been that person for me, as have many others. Both of my children have helped in so many ways too. When they sit next to me and cuddle, give me hugs and kisses, my daughter's gentle touch on my hand or face, her insistence on sleeping next to me, these gifts of touch bring me healing. The many hours I spent sitting with my son reading to him over the years kept my mind off of my cancer and on what was more important. Each time someone reaches out to me in love and helpfulness, I recognize it as a gift from God, reminding me of His trustworthiness.

During my second cancer fight, I had a conversation with my oncologist about all the different cancer diagnoses in my family. He said, "I think there ought to be a limit to the number of cancers in a family and the number of cancers in an individual person. But," and he paused to look up, "I am not sure who to talk to about that." I answered, "All I know is that I worship a God who makes masterpieces out of messes like this." I did not understand why all of these cancer battles were happening to me and my family at the same time. However, I knew it was an exercise in trust. In spite of the difficult road I was traveling, I knew there was a Sovereign God who loved me and was right beside me. The more I get to know who He is, the less what is happening around me matters. He is teaching me to change my grasping, controlling stance to one of openness and trust. As I walked incredibly hard paths, I knew the Lord was right beside me. I could depend on Him to keep me from dangers I could not see. He carried me when it was too difficult to go alone. Like the classic "Footprints in the Sand" poem I realized when it was too difficult for me to go alone, He was carrying me. Like the 23rd Psalm says, "Yea though I walk thru the valley of the shadow of death, thou art with me, thy rod and thy staff, they comfort me." Verse 4, (KJV).

We can grasp onto God's hand and choose to trust Jesus. There will always be something to worry about, but you can choose to trust in the Lord no matter what.

Yes, we can trust our God who was able to make the Heavens and the Earth. We can shout with the prophet Jeremiah, 32:17 (KJV) "Ah Lord God! Behold, thou who hast made the heaven and the earth by thy great power and by stretched out arm! There is nothing too hard for thee." We can trust in Him because He can do anything. We have the example from the book of Job of a man who endured tremendous hardship. He lost family, wealth, health, and home. Job's friends tried to advise and comfort him, and made mistakes along the way. Nevertheless, Job trusted God through all his troubles and God delivered him.

When we face difficult times in our cancer journey and pause to wonder why, we are to remember God is sovereign over all and that He is trustworthy. Job's response in chapter 42: 2 (KJV) is a good response for us to have too. Job replies, "'I know that thou canst do *every* thing, and that no thought can be withholden from thee."

Yes, we can trust God. He is the Creator of our world, the universe, and He made you. God loves you and cares about you. He wants you to trust Him. And ultimately, He calls us to trust Him with our souls. In September 2011, a very good friend of mine died at the age of 39 to colon cancer. She was strong in her faith and always an encouragement to me. I loved the conversations we would have, and I was privileged to have some extra special ones with her in her last month of life. We had been friends for nine years and never had one disagreement. Even though it was hard to watch her lose her fight, I trusted God to see both of us through this difficult time. I trusted that her illness and death was part of His greater plan. I saw her just hours before she died, and said goodbye and thanked her for her friendship. My other parting words to my dear friend were, "remember how much God loves you. You have to hold onto that—He loves you so much!" She held on to her faith and trusted her savior to the end. We need to trust in God and His incredible mercy and love to the end. God has given us the promise of life beyond death, through the resurrection power of His son, Jesus Christ. Jesus shed his blood on the cross, died and was resurrected on the third day. He is in Heaven and is our intercessor. I know that when my friend died Jesus welcomed her with open arms. I have the hope and assurance from the promise of resurrection through Jesus Christ that I will see my friend again when He welcomes me home.

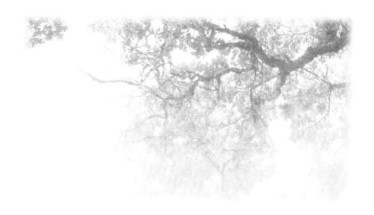

LESSON 7

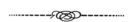

Perspective

Perspective is how we look at things. Perspectives shape who we are and how we deal with our situations. Two people with the same cancer diagnosis could have completely different perspectives. They could have a perspective of acceptance versus denial; of "absolute worst thing that has happened to me" versus "another challenge in life"; a "bump in the road" versus "the end of the road." During my breast cancer treatments I was feeling very low. I received a call from my Pastor. I shared with him some of my feelings. After I finished venting, he gave me the following verse to hang onto: "This is the day which the Lord hath made; we will rejoice and be glad in it." Psalm 118:24 (KJV). He reminded me that despite our circumstances, we should still be thankful for things that we often take for granted. This changed my perspective. Instead of feeling low and despondent, I was able to rise above my depression and remember I was still alive and that hope still abounds, that I did not need to dwell on the negatives, but look for positives to change my outlook. That one simple redirection gave me the new perspective I needed. I proceeded to have a good day, and many good days after that, despite what I was going through. And you can too.

We have a choice of how we live the day. We can fill it with fear, worry, regrets, sorrow, and unhappiness or with praise, thankfulness and kindness. There are certainly plenty of reasons available to explain why we feel the former. The truth is, some days we are so tired, there seems to be no other way to feel. Yet, at the end of that day, what have we accomplished? Are we proud of the way we spent it? Everyone has down days. Anyone who knows me certainly knows I have had my share. I am not saying we have to be upbeat and happy every day. However, it is to our benefit and our loved ones to be positive and productive as much as possible. Give yourself permission to be down and acknowledge it for what it is. One verse that helped me was from Proverbs 18:14 (NIV), "A man's spirit sustains him in sickness, but a crushed spirit who can bear?"

Here is a challenge. One of the quickest ways to bring yourself up is to focus on others. Find one good thing to do for someone else each day, regardless of how you feel. Another way to help bring you up is to find one thing to do for you that will make you smile. If you can have a good day, do. These actions helped me get through the very difficult nine months between August 2009 and March 2010, when my sister, my mother and myself were all going through cancer treatments. Instead of focusing on my woes, I tried to focus on how I could help myself and someone else each day.

Building positive perspective includes living in the moment. By living in the moment, I mean, stop thinking about what is going to happen a year from now, a month, week, or even much about tomorrow. Instead of worrying about the future, focus on here and now, this day, this moment. When life is intense, try breaking your day into increments of 15-60 minutes. This will help you get through the rough times. Be aware of what is happening in the moment. We must live each day we are given to the fullest possible. Strive to end the day with the satisfaction that it was not wasted. It does not have to be a monumental achievement. Set the goal to make a positive difference in one person's life, and you will have succeeded. Tell people you love them. Enjoy your time with them. Every day in life is a gift, and we must embrace it as if it is our last. Spend time building your legacy. You have some time to make or preserve memories, to write letters to loved ones. You have the gift of NOW. That is why it is called the present. Live in the present, and enjoy it thoroughly. To see what the Bible has to say about this, read Ecclesiastes 7:14; 9:7-10; 11:9-10. Present pleasures are God's good gifts. This is how we learn to number our days. How are we going to spend our last few days? Let us ask God for the wisdom to spend them wisely.

The whole point for Christians is that existence does not end in death, nor is death final. John 5:24 (NIV), "I tell you the truth, whoever hears my word and believes him who sent me has eternal life and will not be condemned; he has crossed over from death to life," puts eternal life in the present tense. You have it now.

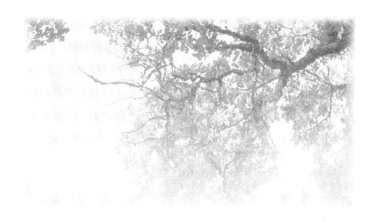

LESSON 8

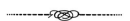

Suffering

As a cancer patient, you are an expert in suffering. We suffer through treatments, tests, needle pokes, and side effects that glue us to our beds or couches some days. I have had days while on the carboplatin drug where I felt like a zombie, so dead tired and out of it. I remember days during treatments for breast cancer when I felt like I had been run over by a semi-truck.

The Israelites during the time of Moses were also experts in suffering. They were enslaved to the Egyptians, made to work very hard building, even forced to make their own bricks. I got the chance while in Mexico to see how to make bricks by hand. It is hard, backbreaking work, digging, making a messy mixture of water, clay and straw, and then putting them in frames. It takes days to make a batch of brick, as they dry out in the sun. When Moses first tried to free God's people, their conditions got worse. The Pharaoh thought them lazy (obviously not understanding the job they had to do) and told them they had to go find their own straw now and still complete the same amount of daily work. The Israelites were suffering greatly under slavery in Egypt. God recognized and was concerned with their suffering. Although they were beaten and discouraged, God heard their cries and He saved them. He freed them from their bondage. Exodus, Chapter 2, verses 23-25 (NIV): "The Israelites . . . cry for help . . . went up to God. God heard their groaning . . . and was concerned about them." I took comfort in knowing that God heard their cries and that He was concerned about them. God is concerned about you too. When you are suffering with symptoms from cancer or side effects from the treatments, God hears your groans and cries. As we read on in Exodus, we learn God has a plan to rescue the Israelites. "The Lord said, 'I have indeed seen the misery of my people in Egypt. I have heard them crying out . . . I have come down to rescue them' . . ." Exodus, Chapter 3, verses 7-8a (NIV). We have a God that hears us, sees us, is concerned about us and is mighty to save us. We can trust Him that He has a plan for our lives too.

There have been many times while in my misery, I cry out to the Lord, and He responds by sending people my way. Some come to give me a hug. Some come with a meal, loaf of bread, or cookies. Maybe they pay me a visit in person, or just a phone call to chat. Email messages and responses to my blog help to lift my day. Each response is another reassurance from the Holy Spirit that God hears me and loves me still.

As Christians, we should not be surprised if we encounter trials that cause us suffering. Peter writes about suffering for being a Christian. He reminds us that suffering can be a good thing, something that we can rejoice in because through our suffering God reveals His glory. See 1 Peter 4:12-13 (KJV),

> Beloved, think it not strange concerning the fiery trial which is to try you, as though some strange thing happened unto you: But rejoice, inasmuch as ye are partakers of Christ's sufferings; that, when his glory shall be revealed, ye may be glad also with exceeding joy.

In the first chapter of James, the author gives instructions on how to behave when we are facing trials and temptations. He provides a perspective that is unique from most of the world. Instead of lamenting and crying out, "woe is me", he says in verse 2 (NIV): "Consider it pure joy, my brothers, whenever you face trials of many kinds." So the next time you go in the chemo room, give out a big "Yippee!" Well, maybe not, but remember that in your suffering there is an unseen spiritual battle where God is working to bring glory to Himself. Find joy in the Holy Spirit that you are a part of this. We can strive to take the focus away from our ailments, and think about God's glory instead. Romans 8:18 (KJV), "For I reckon that the sufferings of this present time are not worthy to be compared with the glory which shall be revealed in us."

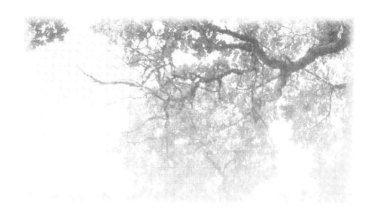

LESSON 9

Sorrow, Loss & Loneliness

I n September 2011, I went to my dear friend's memorial service. It was a hard day for me. I lost a very good friend and with that loss comes a feeling that I am not as okay as I used to be. When someone you love dearly and who loved you in return leaves, we can be left feeling unloved. And yet, this is a perfect time to turn to our loving Heavenly Father, who has so much love for us. I found comfort in the scriptures read at her service.

John chapter 14, verses 1-3 (KJV), "Let not your heart be troubled: ye believe in God, believe also in me. In my Father's house there are many mansions: if it were not so, I would have told you. I go to prepare a place for you, I will come again, and receive you unto myself; that where I am, there ye may be also." These verses reassured me that my friend was in her heavenly dwelling and that when I die, I will get to see her again. We can hold onto this promise of resurrection that is ours through Christ Jesus.

Verses from Psalm 23 really hit home with me and confirmed to me how God fulfills his promises and is always right by our side.

The last two verses of Jude were read at my friend's service, and they tell us about how Jesus will present us to the Father with great joy. Verses 24-25 (KJV), "Now unto him that is able to keep you from falling, and to present you faultless before the presence of his glory with exceeding joy, to the only wise God our Savior, be glory and majesty, dominion and power, both now and ever. Amen." Since Jesus is our propitiation for our sins, we can appear before the Father without fault. Even in our sorrow, we can find joy in this promise!

Sections from Romans 8 were read at her funeral. Reminders that we are children of God, of our spirit of adoption, and that nothing can separate us from the love of God. When I reread Romans chapter 8 again, I hear the author speaking this with such authority and emphasis, shouting it at the crowds. "We are more than conquerors through him that loved us!" Romans 8:37 (KJV) And nothing can "separate us from the love of God, which is in Christ Jesus our Lord!" verse 39 (KJV) Not death, not life, nothing that is now, nothing to come, not cancer, not powers . . . NOTHING CAN SEPARATE US FROM GOD's LOVE! Let's cling to these truths.

My friend did die. I grieve the loss, and yet I know, she is with our Lord and Savior, Jesus Christ. Not even death can separate us from His love. And we know that all things are made new in Christ Jesus. When I saw her in my dream the night after she died, she was made new again, healthy and spunky. We can trust in Christ's promises. This is our reassurance in His resurrection—the Easter promise—the gift of eternal life.

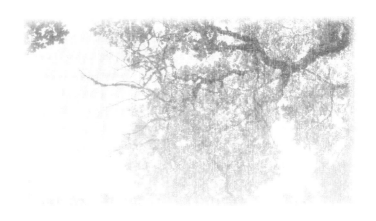

LESSON 10

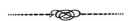

Gratitude

An "attitude of gratitude." How do we cultivate an "attitude of gratitude" in the midst of all that we are going through as cancer patients? How does the Bible apply to this? The Bible has much to say about being thankful and offering sacrifices of thanksgiving. The Bible also reminds us of all God has done for us. How can we not embrace His goodness with gratitude?

Let's start with the basics and go back to the beginning of time. Read the creation story in Genesis 1–3. In the beginning, God created the heavens and the earth. As you read the first two chapters, think about all the beauty of nature around us created by God and thank Him for it. Feel the warmth of the sun. Breathe the atmosphere he made so life on earth can exist. Check out how the animals behave. Note how they live their lives, trusting in God's goodness to provide for their needs. Be aware of all the basic necessities that God created and how He has thought of how every detail works in our bodies. Thanking God for the basics helps us to put our trials into perspective.

Now let us jump to the end of Job, chapters 38-41. Here God gives a first-hand account of what He did and is capable of, reminding us of His sovereignty. If I think about it just a minute, I feel myself overwhelmed by his knowledge and wisdom, of how powerful He is and what He is capable of doing. I cannot begin to fathom His greatness and cannot help but be overcome with thankfulness. The natural response is gratitude, being thankful for His grand creation and that we are a part of it. How easy it is to forget that each new sunrise and sunset is a gift.

Creating a "things to be thankful for" list is another way to develop an attitude of gratitude. It can also help you stay centered in the midst of chaos and tough times, changing your focus off yourself. I remember one September day in 2009, I went with my mom to her doctor's appointment. This was shortly after her breast cancer diagnosis. The doctor was giving her the news that she would have to go through all the same chemotherapy drugs that I had gone through three years before, plus a few more. Mom was quite unhappy about it. I could feel the stress and tension in the room. It seemed like the news just kept getting worse and worse. In the back of my mind, I was concerned for my own health too. To combat the downward spiral of emotions and feelings, I pulled out a piece of paper and started making a list of 10 people I am thankful for and 10 things I am thankful for. This got my Mom's and the doctor's attention and they wanted to know what I was doing, so I told them. This simple action lifted all of us into a more positive place, and we found the strength to complete the appointment. Sometimes it may be hard to come up with 10 reasons to be thankful, but there is always something. Starting with basic provisions like a roof over your head or a bed to sleep in can get you going. There may be a friend or family member for whom you are particularly thankful. Your list does not have to include all grandiose items. It can be just as effective to name simple things like enjoying a chocolate or cup of coffee. When you start your list you will be surprised at how easy it is to come up with 10 things. This exercise changes our perspective, allows us to remember that even though some things are not the way you want them to be, there is plenty to be thankful for. Let us remember our heavenly Father has promised the biggest gift ever, eternal life in Him. 2 Corinthians 9:15 (KJV) "Thanks be unto God for his unspeakable gift!" Thanking Him for that alone may lift our spirits.

Even as we suffer and face death, we can rest assured that God is sovereign. Jesus Christ has completed the work for our salvation. I Corinthians 15:57 (NIV) says, "But thanks be to God! He gives us victory through our Lord Jesus Christ." What an incredible gift! God directs us to be thankful to Him. Over and over again in the scriptures we can find passages calling us to be thankful. Be thankful for who God is and what He has done for us. Thinking about the rest of the world, about bringing Christ into the world through prayers and missions, especially seeing the gospel in countries where it used to be outlawed really shows us how much He is at work. It is so amazing what He has done for us and what He continues to do!

In Colossians 3:15 (KJV) Paul calls us to be thankful, "And let the peace of God rule in your hearts, to the which also ye are called in one body and be ye thankful." One of the gifts of the Holy Spirit is peace. When we are privileged to feel peace, even in the midst of our struggles and tribulations, this is a gift for which to be thankful.

1 Thessalonians 5:18 (KJV) "In every thing give thanks: for this is the will of God in Christ Jesus concerning you." Giving thanks in all circumstances can be hard, especially with the road us as cancer patients often have to travel. Yet, a thankful heart makes such a big difference especially when going through difficult times. Giving thanks to God for He is good is a great exercise for our heart. It reminds our broken hearts how much God loves us. Psalm 107:1 (KJV) "Give thanks unto the Lord, for He is good; for His mercy endureth for ever." I recall a time after one of my friends died of metastatic breast cancer, and I saw her husband and two young sons. I was about to begin my second battle with cancer. At that point, it was hard to find the words to bring comfort. I could only try to point to our rock we cling to in the midst of great personal loss and muster the words, "God is still good."

In the Bible, David sets us a high example. Young David, even when being pursued by his enemies, praised the Lord. He wrote songs of praise that are being used to this day. Reading the Psalms and singing some that have been put to song in modern day can fill our hearts with gratitude.

We know that as we undergo our cancer journeys, Christ is leading us to victory. Our stories can serve as a witness, encouraging others to draw closer to Him.

Finally, in 2 Corinthians 2:14 (NIV) Paul sums it up for us, "But thanks be to God, who always leads us in triumphal procession in Christ and through us spreads everywhere the fragrance of the knowledge of Him."

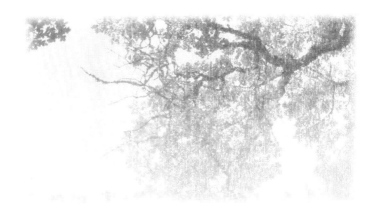

LESSON 11

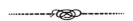

Wisdom

Wisdom is knowing the right thing to do in a circumstance and doing it. Simply put, it is being able to apply knowledge appropriately. James 3 defines two types of wisdom. One is a worldly wisdom that seeds from bitter envy and selfish ambition in our hearts. The other is a wisdom that comes from heaven, "pure; then peace-loving, considerate, submissive, full of mercy and good fruit, impartial and sincere." (James 3:17 NIV) It is easy for us to have a worldly wisdom where we make decisions that are selfish. It is much harder for us to have a heavenly wisdom, one that is pure and not self-seeking. How do we obtain the right kind of wisdom? Where do we get wisdom? We must seek it out. Diving into the scriptures will assist us in receiving the gift of wisdom from God. In the book of Proverbs, you can find a plethora of instruction related to wisdom. Take the time to read it, focusing on the first nine chapters. Proverbs 1:7 (KJV), "The fear of the Lord is the beginning of knowledge: but fools despise wisdom and instruction."

Even though we seek wisdom, God does not promise that He will give us the knowledge of how all things fit together, of how one situation assists another. That is for God to know and decide. He knows how much wisdom we need. We are to trust in Him. We are to live a life of acceptance to what He has given us and praise Him even when we do not know what lies ahead.

God can use our difficult experiences like cancer, to provide wisdom. Ecclesiastes 7:14 (NIV), "When times are good, be happy; but when times are bad, consider: God has made the one as well as the other. Therefore, a man cannot discover anything about his future." If we trust God in good times as well as bad, even though what is occurring does not seem to make sense, we can be sure that it is part of His plan. We may never know why we have been stricken with disease or trials, but we can be sure that God is by our side. When we stop asking "Why?" and start asking "How?" and "What?" He will reveal to us what we need to know. He will show us how to get through the bad with the good. He will show us what we need to do to get through, one day at a time. In this, we become wise in our circumstances. Instead of searching for meaning and reasons why we are in our situation, we need to accept it. When we move to acceptance, we can shift our focus and determination to make the best of it. This results in wisdom. When we face the facts and see life as it is, our wisdom will grow.

God is a giver of gifts. In 1 Kings 3 we can read the story of King Solomon asking God for wisdom. God approached Solomon in a dream, and said, "Ask for whatever you want me to give you." 1 Kings 3:5 (NIV). Solomon asked for a discerning heart to govern the people and know right from wrong. Solomon could have asked for riches, long life or honor, but he asked for wisdom. God was pleased with this request, and gave it to him in abundance. As a bonus, He gave Solomon riches and honor too. James 1:5 encourages us to ask God for wisdom.

What do we do with the wisdom God has revealed to us? We should take the wisdom we have learned and our unique perspective and share it with others. Pass along to them the secrets to a successful life in unusual circumstances. Share with them the joy they can have when they put their trust in God and strive to do His will. Open up with others who are going through similar circumstances and empathize with them. We have all been down and will have our down days. Having an empathetic friend is invaluable. Help each other to not continuously dwell on the negatives. There are positives in all situations, so find them and thank God for them. Share the peace of Christ that is in you with others. Christ has already obtained victory for us. This is the good news. Let's share the good news of the Gospel.

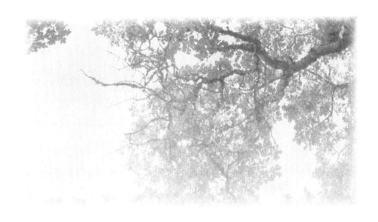

LESSON 12

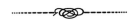

Facing Death & Dying with Hope

All of our lives will eventually end in death. Death is feared and ignored, the word itself is avoided in our culture. Yet we do face death when we have a diagnosis of cancer. Often we are healed and go back to living our lives with valuable lessons learned and the hope that we will not have to face it again. For some, though, the cancer is really going to be the end of our lives. This is where the hope we find in the scriptures shifts from physical healing, to the hope of eternal life in Christ after our death. Remember John 3:16 (KJV),

"For God so loved the world, that He gave his only begotten Son, that whosoever believeth in him shall not perish, but have everlasting life."

Our hope is in the Lord Jesus Christ. Jesus was resurrected from the dead on the third day. You can read the story in each of the four gospels. He fulfilled God's plan for the salvation of our souls. Jesus shows us the path of life. Because of Jesus and what He did, we do not have to be abandoned in our graves. We can have the gift of eternal life. Jesus' body did not see decay because He arose from the dead and lives, seated at the right hand of God. He is our advocate in Heaven.

When Jesus knew the end was near what did He do? How did He spend that time? For those answers, we look to the Gospels of Matthew, Mark, Luke and John. From these passages, we know that Jesus understands our suffering. He also knew his death was imminent. When faced with death, He chose to follow God's will, being obedient, all the way to the end. When we are faced with life's uncertainties, we can strive to be obedient to God too. To hear what his last words to the disciples were, read John chapters 14–17.

When Jesus was troubled, he took it to his Heavenly Father in prayer. Because Jesus is the propitiation for our sins, we can also turn to God in prayer during our trying times. In His final hours, Jesus prayed very hard to His Heavenly Father. Luke 22: 44b (KJV), "And being in agony he prayed more earnestly: and His sweat was as it were great drops of blood falling down to the ground." In Matthew 26:38 (NLT) we hear Jesus say, "'My soul is crushed with grief to the point of death. Stay here and keep watch with Me.'" Have you ever felt so alone and sorrow filled? I know I have had moments in my cancer journeys, scary dark lonely moments, but not to the point of death. Jesus then goes a short distance away from his friends and prays on His own three different times. Each time He asks His Father if it is possible to take the cup of suffering away, yet each time Jesus emphasizes His willingness to do whatever is His Father's will, even if that will includes him suffering and dying on the cross. When I think of Jesus shedding His blood for me on the cross, the nails driven through his wrists and feet, I think the needle pokes and test tubes of blood I have given are too small even to compare.

Although life is a gift to be treasured, it is not easy. The end of life is no exception. We have to build up the spiritual muscles to endure to the end. We know that God, in His Goodness, gives us even more than life. He gives us the promises of eternal life in His Son Jesus. Read 1 Peter 1:3-9. The beautiful comfort and promises in this passage says it all. Jesus offers us a living hope through His resurrection. We suffer now in grief and trials so that our faith may be proved genuine. The goal of our faith is the salvation of our souls.

Jesus points to God's creation to show that in death, more life is created. John 12:24 (NLT) says, "The truth is, a kernel of wheat must be planted in the soil. Unless it dies it will be alone-a single seed. But its death will produce many new kernels—a plentiful harvest of new lives." I like this gardening analogy and it gives me hope to think that when a plant dies it goes to seed and those seeds make thousands of plants grow.

At some point in our spiritual journey, may we arrive to the place where we can say with Paul, as he did in his second letter to the Corinthians 5:8 (KJV), "We are confident, I say, and willing rather to be absent from the body, and to be present with the Lord." At times, I do feel like I have reached this point. Yet a huge part of me is sad to think of things I will miss out on earth. I have two beautiful children that I would like to watch grow up. I have a husband I love and with whom I want to grow old. Yet, if this is not what is meant to be, I have to stay focused on knowing that what comes after this life is even more glorious. There are few details available about what Heaven is like. I think that is a big reason why it is difficult to look forward to going to Heaven. The unknown is hard.

See Revelations chapter 19, and chapter 21-22 for what the Bible has to say about Heaven. When you know someone really well, you might look forward to going to his or her house. The more we get to know Jesus and our Heavenly Father, the more we are able to trust in Him, and the more comfortable we may become with joining Him in Heaven. Reading the Bible is a great way to get to know God and his heart. The more we know God, the more comfortable we will feel in going home to our Heavenly Father.

We know there is a gift after this life. 2 Corinthians 5:5 (NLT) "God himself has prepared us for this, and as a guarantee He has given us His Holy Spirit." This is the blessed assurance referred to in hymns.

In 2 Corinthians chapter 4, verses 14-15 Paul reminds us of the hope of resurrection we have because of Jesus. By God's grace, it brings glory to God when we embrace this hope and be thankful. Because of this incredible gift, we live what we have left of our lives to please God and bring Him glory.

How can a mother of two young children face cancer? Because I do not face it alone. I don't have to be in charge. The journey through cancer has made me more and more dependent upon God as the illusion of control is wiped away. God loves us so much. We are His children. He has already done all of the work through Jesus' death on the cross and His resurrection. As the creator and author of our faith; He started the work and He has competed the work. We are creatures in a fallen world. The cancer that is eating at our bodies is just another representation of what is wrong in this world since sin entered at the fall in the Garden of Eden. We are not our cancer. We are loved children of God.

John 11:25-26 (KJV), "Jesus said unto her, "I am the resurrection, and the life: he that believeth in me, though he were dead, yet shall he live: And whosoever liveth and believeth in me shall never die. Believest thou this?"

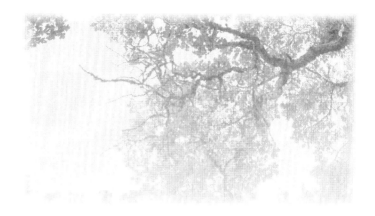

EPILOGUE

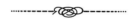

As I complete this book, my sister, Debbie, and I are each facing another battle with cancer. She had surgery to remove a brain tumor, with radiation and more chemotherapy to look forward to afterwards. I find myself once again in the unknown—knowing my tumor markers are high, scans showing cancer and chemotherapy appointments to find out what is next. As we battle cancer together continuously, we hold onto the promises of our Lord for life after death. We still go through all the range of emotions, including anger, fear and sadness. 2 Corinthians 1:9 (KJV) "But we had the sentence of death in ourselves, that we should not trust in ourselves, but in God which raiseth the dead." God has been good to see us through many difficult trials, restoring our bodies to health, giving us breaks between treatments. We have the gift of going through it together. We both feel every day we have on earth with our children and husbands and families is a gift. For these things, we can offer the sacrifice of thanksgiving and fill our hearts with gratitude to our Creator.

I just had my 40th birthday. I have made it this far by the grace of God. Regardless of what the future brings, we can draw hope from Jesus, because He is the one with the last word. He has demonstrated the power of resurrection for us all. In Him we are offered new life. Debbie's beautiful testament when she told me about her brain tumor, "the peace of Christ is all that is holding me together."

It is our hope and prayer that regardless of the stage or progression of your disease, as you read these lessons you are awakened by the Holy Spirit to the comfort found in the Holy Scriptures, and a desire within you to read the bible is renewed. If so, this too is a gift from God to be treasured. If the cancer you have experienced draws you closer to Him, as it has my sister and I, consider yourself blessed. The more difficulties we go through in life, the more the Bible has to say to us and the more it makes sense. If this book has helped to open your eyes and your ears to what the Bible has to say, then Praise be to the Lord for his kindness!

If reading this book has renewed your interest in reading the bible . . . if it has brought you hope, encouragement and comfort, then you make my joy complete. Most importantly, if this book brings glory to God, then mission accomplished.

"Now unto God and our Father be glory for ever and ever. Amen." Philippians 4:20 (KJV)

"The grace of our Lord Jesus Christ be with you all. Amen." Philippians 4:23 (KJV)

"And the peace of God, which passeth all understanding, shall keep your hearts and minds through Christ Jesus." Philippians 4:7 (KJV)

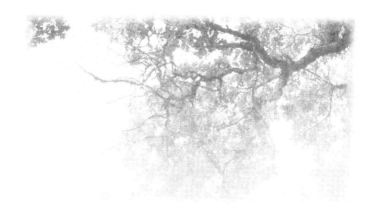

ABOUT THE AUTHOR

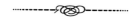

J anet Gaston has battled cancer four times in the last seven years. Each time, her faith and dependence upon our Heavenly Father grew. Janet lives with her husband and their two children in Oregon. She is a member of Zion Lutheran church and two cancer support groups.

CPSIA information can be obtained
at www.ICGtesting.com
Printed in the USA
FSOW01n2231011215
13903FS

9 781449 799243